28-DAY PREVENTION ANTI-INFLAMMATORY COOKBOOK

4-Week Meal Plans to Heal the Immune System and Restore Overall Health

Dr Lily Morgan

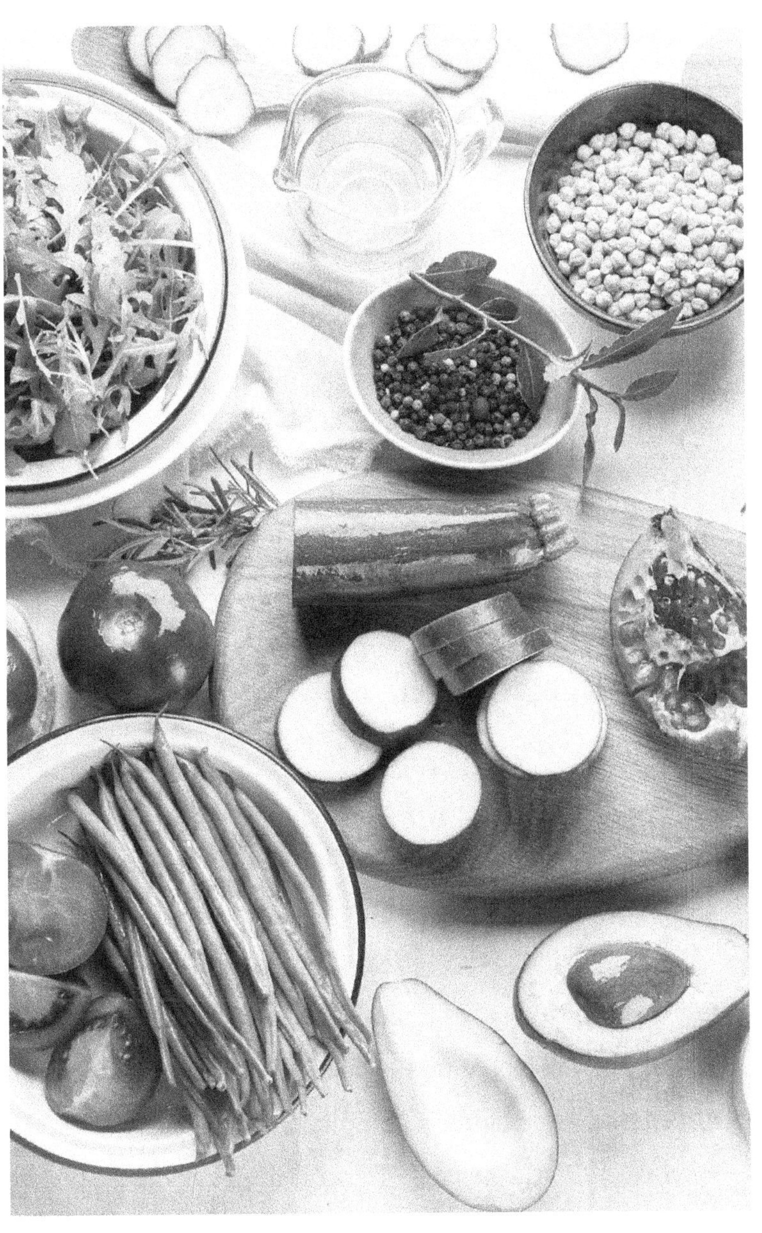

TABLE OF CONTENTS

INTRODUCTION

Inflammation is a natural response of the body's immune system to protect and heal itself from injury or infection. It is a complex biological process involving various cells, chemicals, and immune responses. While acute inflammation is a necessary and beneficial part of the body's defense mechanism, chronic inflammation can have detrimental effects on overall health.

In recent years, scientific research has uncovered the link between chronic inflammation and the development of various diseases such as cardiovascular diseases, diabetes, obesity, autoimmune disorders, and even certain types of cancer. Chronic inflammation occurs when the immune system becomes overactive or fails to shut down after an initial injury or infection. This sustained inflammatory response can damage healthy tissues and organs, leading to the onset and progression of chronic diseases.

Understanding the Importance of an Anti-Inflammatory Diet

The good news is that we have the power to modulate and control inflammation through lifestyle choices, particularly through our diet. An anti-inflammatory diet focuses on consuming foods that help reduce inflammation in the body and promote overall health and well-being. By making conscious choices about what we eat, we can potentially mitigate the risks associated with chronic inflammation and improve our overall quality of life.

The 28-Day Prevention Anti-Inflammatory Cookbook is designed to provide you with a comprehensive guide to adopting an anti-inflammatory diet. It offers a diverse range of delicious and nutritious recipes that incorporate key anti-inflammatory ingredients, allowing you to embark on a culinary journey that promotes both health and flavor.

Benefits of the 28-Day Prevention Anti-Inflammatory Cookbook

This cookbook is not just another fad diet or a temporary solution. It is a lifestyle approach aimed at long-term health and wellness. By following the recipes and meal plans outlined in this cookbook, you can experience a multitude of benefits, including:

Reduced Inflammation: The recipes in this cookbook are carefully crafted to include ingredients that possess anti-inflammatory properties. These ingredients can help counteract chronic inflammation, promoting a healthier and more balanced immune response.

Disease Prevention: Chronic inflammation has been linked to the development of various diseases. By adopting an anti-inflammatory diet, you may reduce the risk of developing conditions such as heart disease, diabetes, arthritis, and certain cancers.

Weight Management: Inflammation can disrupt the body's metabolism and contribute to weight gain and obesity. The recipes in this cookbook are designed to support weight management by incorporating whole, nutrient-dense foods and emphasizing portion control.

Enhanced Nutritional Intake: The recipes in this cookbook prioritize the inclusion of nutrient-rich ingredients, such as fruits, vegetables, whole grains, lean proteins, and healthy fats. By following these recipes, you can improve your overall nutritional intake and ensure that your body receives the essential vitamins, minerals, and antioxidants it needs to function optimally.

Improved Digestion: Many of the recipes in this cookbook incorporate ingredients that support healthy digestion, such as fiber-rich foods, probiotics, and gut-friendly ingredients. A healthy digestive system plays a crucial role in overall well-being and can contribute to reduced inflammation.

How to Use This Cookbook

This cookbook is organized in a user-friendly manner to help you navigate through the 28-day journey of adopting an anti-inflammatory diet. Here are some key features and tips to make the most of this resource:

Meal Plans: The 28-Day Meal Plan section provides a comprehensive guide to your daily meals throughout the four weeks. Each week is carefully structured to ensure a balanced and varied diet, while also incorporating anti-inflammatory ingredients. You can follow the meal plans as they are or mix and match the recipes according to your preferences.

Recipe Diversity: The cookbook offers a wide range of recipes for breakfast, lunch, dinner, snacks, appetizers, desserts, and smoothies. This diversity ensures that you won't get bored with repetitive meals and allows you to explore new flavors and culinary experiences.

Ingredient Substitutions: Feel free to make ingredient substitutions based on your dietary preferences, allergies, or ingredient availability. However, keep in mind that certain ingredients are specifically chosen for their anti-inflammatory properties, so try to maintain the core principles of the recipes.

Nutritional Information: Each recipe is accompanied by nutritional information, including calorie count, macronutrient breakdown, and key vitamins and minerals. This information can be helpful for tracking your nutrient intake and maintaining a balanced diet.

Cooking Tips: Throughout the cookbook, you will find cooking tips and suggestions to help you make the most of each recipe. These tips may include ingredient preparation techniques, alternative cooking methods, or suggestions for enhancing flavors.

By immersing yourself in the 28-Day Prevention Anti-Inflammatory Cookbook, you are taking an important step towards improving your health and well-being. The recipes within this cookbook are not only nourishing but also flavorful and satisfying. Embrace this journey, savor each bite, and embrace the positive changes that an anti-inflammatory lifestyle can bring.

Remember, this cookbook is just the beginning. The knowledge and habits you develop throughout these 28 days can be carried forward to create a sustainable and healthy approach to eating for years to come. Let's embark on this culinary adventure together and experience the transformative power of an anti-inflammatory diet.

Chapter 1: 28-Day Meal Plan

Week 1: Daily Meal Plan

Day 1:

Breakfast: Berry Chia Seed Pudding

Lunch: Greek Salad with Grilled Chicken

Dinner: Baked Salmon with Dill and Lemon

Snack: Roasted Red Pepper Hummus with Crudites

Dessert: Mixed Berry Parfait with Greek Yogurt

Smoothie: Green Detox Smoothie with Spinach and Pineapple

Day 2:

Breakfast: Avocado Toast with Smoked Salmon

Lunch: Quinoa and Roasted Vegetable Salad

Dinner: Grilled Chicken Breast with Roasted Vegetables

Snack: Greek Yogurt and Cucumber Dip

Dessert: Dark Chocolate Avocado Mousse

Smoothie: Berry Blast Smoothie with Almond Milk

Day 3:

Breakfast: Quinoa Breakfast Bowl with Mixed Berries

Lunch: Salmon and Avocado Salad with Lemon Vinaigrette

Dinner: Quinoa and Black Bean Stuffed Peppers

Snack: Baked Kale Chips with Sea Salt

Dessert: Baked Apples with Cinnamon and Walnuts

Smoothie: Mango Turmeric Smoothie with Coconut Water

Day 4:

Breakfast: Veggie Omelette with Spinach and Mushrooms

Lunch: Chickpea and Vegetable Curry

Dinner: Mediterranean Grilled Shrimp Skewers

Snack: Smoked Salmon Roll-Ups with Cream Cheese

Dessert: Coconut Chia Pudding with Mango

Smoothie: Chocolate Banana Protein Smoothie

Day 5:

Breakfast: Overnight Oats with Almond Milk and Blueberries

Lunch: Turkey Lettuce Wraps with Hummus

Dinner: Sweet Potato and Kale Curry

Snack: Caprese Skewers with Balsamic Glaze

Dessert: Almond Flour Blueberry Muffins

Smoothie: Pineapple and Ginger Smoothie with Flaxseeds

Day 6:

Breakfast: Sweet Potato Hash with Poached Eggs

Lunch: Roasted Vegetable and Goat Cheese Tart

Dinner: Herb-Roasted Turkey Breast with Green Beans

Snack: Zucchini Fritters with Yogurt Sauce

Dessert: Banana Ice Cream with Almond Butter Swirl

Smoothie: Creamy Avocado and Spinach Smoothie

Day 7:

Breakfast: Green Smoothie Bowl with Spinach and Banana

Lunch: Asian Noodle Salad with Peanut Dressing

Dinner: Lentil and Vegetable Casserole

Snack: Spicy Roasted Chickpeas

Dessert: Lemon Poppy Seed Energy Balls

Smoothie: Blueberry Almond Butter Smoothie

Week 2: Daily Meal Plan

Day 8:

Breakfast: Buckwheat Pancakes with Fresh Fruit Compote

Lunch: Mediterranean Quinoa Stuffed Bell Peppers

Dinner: Spaghetti Squash with Tomato Basil Sauce

Snack: Guacamole with Baked Tortilla Chips

Dessert: Raspberry Coconut Bars

Smoothie: Tropical Mango Pineapple Smoothie

Day 9:

Breakfast: Mediterranean Egg Muffins with Feta and Olives

Lunch: Lentil Soup with Turmeric and Ginger

Dinner: Ginger and Garlic Glazed Tofu with Stir-Fried Vegetables

Snack: Stuffed Mushrooms with Spinach and Feta

Dessert: Pumpkin Pie Chia Pudding

Smoothie: Beet and Berry Smoothie with Greek Yogurt

Day 10:

Breakfast: Turmeric Golden Milk Smoothie

Lunch: Caprese Quinoa Salad with Balsamic Glaze

Dinner: Beef and Broccoli Stir-Fry

Snack: Buffalo Cauliflower Bites

Dessert: Berry Crumble with Oat Topping

Smoothie: Peanut Butter and Banana Smoothie

Day 11:

Breakfast: Banana Walnut Muffins with Oat Flour

Lunch: Greek Salad with Grilled Chicken

Dinner: Baked Salmon with Dill and Lemon

Snack: Roasted Red Pepper Hummus with Crudites

Dessert: Mixed Berry Parfait with Greek Yogurt

Smoothie: Green Detox Smoothie with Spinach and

Pineapple

Day 12:

Breakfast: Avocado Toast with Smoked Salmon

Lunch: Quinoa and Roasted Vegetable Salad

Dinner: Grilled Chicken Breast with Roasted Vegetables

Snack: Greek Yogurt and Cucumber Dip

Dessert: Dark Chocolate Avocado Mousse

Smoothie: Berry Blast Smoothie with Almond Milk

Day 13:

Breakfast: Quinoa Breakfast Bowl with Mixed Berries

Lunch: Salmon and Avocado Salad with Lemon

Vinaigrette

Dinner: Quinoa and Black Bean Stuffed Peppers

Snack: Baked Kale Chips with Sea Salt

Dessert: Baked Apples with Cinnamon and Walnuts

Smoothie: Mango Turmeric Smoothie with Coconut Water

Day 14:

Breakfast: Veggie Omelette with Spinach and Mushrooms

Lunch: Chickpea and Vegetable Curry

Dinner: Mediterranean Grilled Shrimp Skewers

Snack: Smoked Salmon Roll-Ups with Cream Cheese

Dessert: Coconut Chia Pudding with Mango

Smoothie: Chocolate Banana Protein Smoothie

Week 3: Daily Meal Plan

Day 15:

Breakfast: Overnight Oats with Almond Milk and Blueberries

Lunch: Turkey Lettuce Wraps with Hummus

Dinner: Sweet Potato and Kale Curry

Snack: Caprese Skewers with Balsamic Glaze

Dessert: Almond Flour Blueberry Muffins

Smoothie: Pineapple and Ginger Smoothie with Flaxseeds

Day 16:

Breakfast: Sweet Potato Hash with Poached Eggs

Lunch: Roasted Vegetable and Goat Cheese Tart

Dinner: Herb-Roasted Turkey Breast with Green Beans

Snack: Zucchini Fritters with Yogurt Sauce

Dessert: Banana Ice Cream with Almond Butter Swirl

Smoothie: Creamy Avocado and Spinach Smoothie

Day 17:

Breakfast: Green Smoothie Bowl with Spinach and Banana

Lunch: Asian Noodle Salad with Peanut Dressing

Dinner: Lentil and Vegetable Casserole

Snack: Spicy Roasted Chickpeas

Dessert: Lemon Poppy Seed Energy Balls

Smoothie: Blueberry Almond Butter Smoothie

Day 18:

Breakfast: Buckwheat Pancakes with Fresh Fruit Compote

Lunch: Mediterranean Quinoa Stuffed Bell Peppers

Dinner: Spaghetti Squash with Tomato Basil Sauce

Snack: Guacamole with Baked Tortilla Chips

Dessert: Raspberry Coconut Bars

Smoothie: Tropical Mango Pineapple Smoothie

Day 19:

Breakfast: Mediterranean Egg Muffins with Feta and Olives

Lunch: Lentil Soup with Turmeric and Ginger

Dinner: Ginger and Garlic Glazed Tofu with Stir-Fried Vegetables

Snack: Stuffed Mushrooms with Spinach and Feta

Dessert: Pumpkin Pie Chia Pudding

Smoothie: Beet and Berry Smoothie with Greek Yogurt

Day 20:

Breakfast: Turmeric Golden Milk Smoothie

Lunch: Caprese Quinoa Salad with Balsamic Glaze

Dinner: Beef and Broccoli Stir-Fry

Snack: Buffalo Cauliflower Bites

Dessert: Berry Crumble with Oat Topping

Smoothie: Peanut Butter and Banana Smoothie

Day 21:

Breakfast: Banana Walnut Muffins with Oat Flour

Lunch: Greek Salad with Grilled Chicken

Dinner: Baked Salmon with Dill and Lemon

Snack: Roasted Red Pepper Hummus with Crudites

Dessert: Mixed Berry Parfait with Greek Yogurt

Smoothie: Green Detox Smoothie with Spinach and Pineapple

Week 4: Daily Meal Plan

Day 22:

Breakfast: Avocado Toast with Smoked Salmon

Lunch: Quinoa and Roasted Vegetable Salad

Dinner: Grilled Chicken Breast with Roasted Vegetables

Snack: Greek Yogurt and Cucumber Dip

Dessert: Dark Chocolate Avocado Mousse

Smoothie: Berry Blast Smoothie with Almond Milk

Day 23:

Breakfast: Quinoa Breakfast Bowl with Mixed Berries

Lunch: Salmon and Avocado Salad with Lemon Vinaigrette

Dinner: Quinoa and Black Bean Stuffed Peppers

Snack: Baked Kale Chips with Sea Salt

Dessert: Baked Apples with Cinnamon and Walnuts

Smoothie: Mango Turmeric Smoothie with Coconut Water

Day 24:

Breakfast: Veggie Omelette with Spinach and Mushrooms

Lunch: Chickpea and Vegetable Curry

Dinner: Mediterranean Grilled Shrimp Skewers

Snack: Smoked Salmon Roll-Ups with Cream Cheese

Dessert: Coconut Chia Pudding with Mango

Smoothie: Chocolate Banana Protein Smoothie

Day 25:

Breakfast: Overnight Oats with Almond Milk and Blueberries

Lunch: Turkey Lettuce Wraps with Hummus

Dinner: Sweet Potato and Kale Curry

Snack: Caprese Skewers with Balsamic Glaze

Dessert: Almond Flour Blueberry Muffins

Smoothie: Pineapple and Ginger Smoothie with Flaxseeds

Day 26:

Breakfast: Sweet Potato Hash with Poached Eggs

Lunch: Roasted Vegetable and Goat Cheese Tart

Dinner: Herb-Roasted Turkey Breast with Green Beans

Snack: Zucchini Fritters with Yogurt Sauce

Dessert: Banana Ice Cream with Almond Butter Swirl

Smoothie: Creamy Avocado and Spinach Smoothie

Day 27:

Breakfast: Green Smoothie Bowl with Spinach and Banana

Lunch: Asian Noodle Salad with Peanut Dressing

Dinner: Lentil and Vegetable Casserole

Snack: Spicy Roasted Chickpeas

Dessert: Lemon Poppy Seed Energy Balls

Smoothie: Blueberry Almond Butter Smoothie

Day 28:

Breakfast: Buckwheat Pancakes with Fresh Fruit Compote

Lunch: Mediterranean Quinoa Stuffed Bell Peppers

Dinner: Spaghetti Squash with Tomato Basil Sauce

Snack: Guacamole with Baked Tortilla Chips

Dessert: Raspberry Coconut Bars

Smoothie: Tropical Mango Pineapple Smoothie

Chapter 2: Breakfast Recipes

In this chapter, we will explore a variety of delicious and nutritious breakfast recipes that are not only satisfying but also anti-inflammatory. These recipes will provide you with the energy you need to kickstart your day while supporting your overall health and well-being. So, let's dive in and discover these delightful morning treats!

Berry Chia Seed Pudding

Ingredients:

- 1 cup almond milk
- 3 tablespoons chia seeds
- 1 tablespoon honey or maple syrup
- 1/2 teaspoon vanilla extract
- 1/2 cup mixed berries (strawberries, blueberries, raspberries)

Instructions:

1. In a bowl, combine almond milk, chia seeds, honey or maple syrup, and vanilla extract. Mix well.

2. Let the mixture sit for 10 minutes, stirring occasionally to prevent clumps.

3. Transfer the mixture into a glass or jar and refrigerate overnight or for at least 4 hours.

4. Before serving, top the chia pudding with mixed berries. Enjoy the creamy and fruity goodness!

Avocado Toast with Smoked Salmon

Ingredients:

- 2 slices of whole grain bread, toasted
- 1 ripe avocado
- Juice of 1/2 lemon
- Salt and pepper to taste
- 4 ounces smoked salmon
- Fresh dill, for garnish

Instructions:

1. In a small bowl, mash the ripe avocado with lemon juice, salt, and pepper.

2. Spread the avocado mixture evenly on the toasted bread slices.

3. Top each slice with smoked salmon and garnish with fresh dill.

4. Serve immediately and savor the combination of creamy avocado and flavorful smoked salmon.

Quinoa Breakfast Bowl with Mixed Berries

Ingredients:

- 1/2 cup cooked quinoa
- 1/4 cup almond milk
- 1 tablespoon honey or maple syrup
- 1/4 teaspoon cinnamon
- 1/2 cup mixed berries (strawberries, blueberries, raspberries)
- 2 tablespoons chopped nuts (almonds, walnuts, or pecans)
- Fresh mint leaves, for garnish

Instructions:

1. In a bowl, combine cooked quinoa, almond milk, honey or maple syrup, and cinnamon. Mix well.

2. Gently fold in the mixed berries and chopped nuts.

3. Garnish with fresh mint leaves for a refreshing touch.

4. Enjoy this protein-packed and fiber-rich quinoa breakfast bowl, packed with antioxidants and vitamins.

Veggie Omelette with Spinach and Mushrooms

Ingredients:

- 3 eggs
- 1 tablespoon olive oil
- 1 cup spinach, washed and chopped
- 1/2 cup sliced mushrooms
- Salt and pepper to taste
- Fresh parsley, for garnish

Instructions:

1. In a bowl, beat the eggs and season with salt and pepper.

2. Heat olive oil in a non-stick skillet over medium heat.

3. Add the spinach and mushrooms to the skillet and sauté until wilted.

4. Pour the beaten eggs over the vegetables and cook until the edges start to set.

5. Gently lift the edges of the omelette with a spatula to allow the uncooked eggs to flow underneath.

6. Once the omelette is set but still slightly runny on top, fold it in half.

7. Transfer the omelette to a plate and garnish with fresh parsley.

8. Serve this flavorful and nutrient-rich veggie omelette for a satisfying breakfast.

Overnight Oats with Almond Milk and Blueberries

Ingredients:

- 1/2 cup rolled oats
- 1/2 cup almond milk
- 1 tablespoon chia seeds
- 1 tablespoon honey or maple syrup
- 1/4 teaspoon vanilla extract
- 1/2 cup fresh or frozen blueberries

- 1 tablespoon sliced almonds

Instructions:

1. In a jar or container, combine rolled oats, almond milk, chia seeds, honey or maple syrup, and vanilla extract. Stir well.
2. Add fresh or frozen blueberries to the mixture and gently mix.
3. Cover the jar or container and refrigerate overnight or for at least 4 hours.
4. Before serving, sprinkle sliced almonds on top for added crunch.
5. Enjoy these creamy and nutritious overnight oats that require no cooking.

Sweet Potato Hash with Poached Eggs

Ingredients:

- 1 large sweet potato, peeled and diced
- 1 red bell pepper, diced
- 1 small onion, diced
- 2 tablespoons olive oil

- 1/2 teaspoon paprika
- Salt and pepper to taste
- 4 large eggs
- Fresh cilantro, for garnish

Instructions:

1. In a skillet, heat olive oil over medium heat.
2. Add sweet potato, red bell pepper, and onion to the skillet. Sauté until the sweet potato is tender and lightly browned.
3. Sprinkle paprika, salt, and pepper over the sweet potato mixture and mix well.
4. Create four wells in the hash and crack an egg into each well.
5. Cover the skillet and cook until the eggs are poached to your desired doneness.
6. Garnish with fresh cilantro for a burst of flavor.
7. Serve this hearty sweet potato hash with perfectly poached eggs for a protein-packed breakfast.

Green Smoothie Bowl with Spinach and Banana

Ingredients:

- 1 ripe banana
- 1 cup fresh spinach
- 1/2 cup almond milk
- 1 tablespoon almond butter
- 1 tablespoon honey or maple syrup
- Toppings: sliced banana, chia seeds, granola, coconut flakes

Instructions:

1. In a blender, combine ripe banana, fresh spinach, almond milk, almond butter, and honey or maple syrup. Blend until smooth and creamy.
2. Pour the green smoothie into a bowl.
3. Top with sliced banana, chia seeds, granola, and coconut flakes for added texture and flavor.
4. Enjoy this vibrant and nutrient-packed green smoothie bowl, a perfect way to incorporate greens into your breakfast.

Buckwheat Pancakes with Fresh Fruit Compote

Ingredients:

- 1 cup buckwheat flour
- 1 tablespoon ground flaxseed
- 1 teaspoon baking powder
- 1/2 teaspoon cinnamon
- 1 cup almond milk
- 1 tablespoon honey or maple syrup
- 1 teaspoon vanilla extract
- Fresh fruit compote: mixed berries, sliced peaches, or any desired fruits

Instructions:

1. In a bowl, whisk together buckwheat flour, ground flaxseed, baking powder, and cinnamon.
2. In a separate bowl, combine almond milk, honey or maple syrup, and vanilla extract. Mix well.
3. Pour the wet ingredients into the dry ingredients and stir until just combined.
4. Heat a non-stick skillet or griddle over medium heat and lightly grease with cooking spray or oil.

5. Pour a quarter cup of batter onto the skillet and
    spread it into a circle.

6. Cook until bubbles form on the surface, then flip the
    pancake and cook for another minute.

7. Repeat with the remaining batter to make more
    pancakes.

8. Serve the buckwheat pancakes with a delightful
    fresh fruit compotemade by simmering mixed
    berries or sliced peaches until soft and juicy.

9. Drizzle the fruit compote over the pancakes for a
    burst of fruity sweetness.

10. Enjoy these wholesome and gluten-free buckwheat
    pancakes with a delicious fruit compote for a
    delightful breakfast experience.

Mediterranean Egg Muffins with Feta and Olives

Ingredients:

- 6 large eggs
- 1/4 cup crumbled feta cheese
- 1/4 cup chopped Kalamata olives
- 1/4 cup diced tomatoes

- 2 tablespoons chopped fresh basil
- Salt and pepper to taste

Instructions:

1. Preheat the oven to 350°F (175°C) and lightly grease a muffin tin.
2. In a bowl, beat the eggs and season with salt and pepper.
3. Stir in crumbled feta cheese, chopped Kalamata olives, diced tomatoes, and chopped fresh basil.
4. Pour the egg mixture evenly into the prepared muffin tin.
5. Bake for about 15-18 minutes or until the egg muffins are set and slightly golden.
6. Remove from the oven and let them cool for a few minutes before removing from the muffin tin.
7. Serve these Mediterranean-inspired egg muffins for a protein-packed breakfast that's full of flavor.

Turmeric Golden Milk Smoothie

Ingredients:

- 1 cup unsweetened almond milk

- 1 ripe banana
- 1/2 teaspoon ground turmeric
- 1/2 teaspoon ground cinnamon
- 1/2 teaspoon grated fresh ginger
- 1 tablespoon honey or maple syrup
- 1 tablespoon almond butter
- Ice cubes

Instructions:

1. In a blender, combine almond milk, ripe banana, ground turmeric, ground cinnamon, grated fresh ginger, honey or maple syrup, and almond butter.
2. Add a few ice cubes to the blender for a refreshing and chilled smoothie.
3. Blend until smooth and creamy.
4. Pour into a glass and sprinkle a pinch of ground turmeric or cinnamon on top for an extra pop of color.
5. Sip on this golden milk smoothie and enjoy the soothing and anti-inflammatory benefits of turmeric.

Banana Walnut Muffins with Oat Flour

Ingredients:

- 1 1/2 cups oat flour (made from grinding rolled oats)
- 1/2 cup almond flour
- 1 teaspoon baking powder
- 1/2 teaspoon baking soda
- 1/4 teaspoon salt
- 2 ripe bananas, mashed
- 1/4 cup honey or maple syrup
- 1/4 cup unsweetened applesauce
- 1/4 cup almond milk
- 1 teaspoon vanilla extract
- 1/2 cup chopped walnuts

Instructions:

1. Preheat the oven to 350°F (175°C) and line a muffin tin with paper liners.
2. In a large bowl, whisk together oat flour, almond flour, baking powder, baking soda, and salt.

3. In another bowl, mix mashed bananas, honey or maple syrup, unsweetened applesauce, almond milk, and vanilla extract.
4. Pour the wet ingredients into the dry ingredients and stir until just combined.
5. Fold in the chopped walnuts.
6. Spoon the batter into the prepared muffin tin, filling each liner about three-quarters full.
7. Bake for approximately 18-20 minutes or until a toothpick inserted into the center comes out clean.
8. Allow the muffins to cool in the tin for a few minutes, then transfer them to a wire rack to cool completely.
9. Enjoy these moist and nutty banana walnut muffins as a wholesome and flavorful breakfast treat.

Chapter 3: Lunch Recipes

In this chapter, we will explore a variety of delicious and healthy lunch recipes that are perfect for incorporating into your anti-inflammatory diet. These recipes are designed to provide you with nourishing ingredients and flavors while promoting a balanced and satisfying meal. Let's dive into the mouthwatering lunch options!

Greek Salad with Grilled Chicken

Ingredients:

- 2 boneless, skinless chicken breasts
- 1 tablespoon olive oil
- 1 teaspoon dried oregano
- Salt and pepper, to taste
- 4 cups mixed salad greens
- 1 cup cherry tomatoes, halved
- 1/2 cucumber, sliced
- 1/2 red onion, thinly sliced
- 1/4 cup Kalamata olives
- 1/4 cup crumbled feta cheese

- Juice of 1 lemon

- 2 tablespoons extra-virgin olive oil

Instructions:

1. Preheat the grill to medium-high heat.
2. Brush the chicken breasts with olive oil and sprinkle with dried oregano, salt, and pepper.
3. Grill the chicken for 6-8 minutes per side, or until cooked through. Let it rest for a few minutes, then slice it into thin strips.
4. In a large bowl, combine the salad greens, cherry tomatoes, cucumber, red onion, Kalamata olives, and crumbled feta cheese.
5. In a small bowl, whisk together the lemon juice and extra-virgin olive oil to make the dressing.
6. Drizzle the dressing over the salad and toss to combine.
7. Divide the salad onto plates and top with the grilled chicken strips. Serve and enjoy!

Quinoa and Roasted Vegetable Salad

Ingredients:

- 1 cup quinoa
- 2 cups water
- 1 red bell pepper, diced
- 1 yellow bell pepper, diced
- 1 zucchini, diced
- 1 eggplant, diced
- 1 red onion, thinly sliced
- 3 tablespoons olive oil
- 2 tablespoons balsamic vinegar
- 1 garlic clove, minced
- 1/4 cup chopped fresh basil
- Salt and pepper, to taste

Instructions:

1. Preheat the oven to 400°F (200°C).
2. Rinse the quinoa under cold water and drain.
3. In a medium saucepan, bring the water to a boil. Add the quinoa, reduce heat to low, cover, and simmer for 15-20 minutes, or until the quinoa is

tender and the water is absorbed. Remove from heat and let it cool.

4. Place the diced red bell pepper, yellow bell pepper, zucchini, eggplant, and red onion on a baking sheet. Drizzle with olive oil, balsamic vinegar, and minced garlic. Season with salt and pepper, then toss to coat.

5. Roast the vegetables in the preheated oven for 20-25 minutes, or until they are tender and slightly caramelized.

6. In a large bowl, combine the cooked quinoa, roasted vegetables, and chopped fresh basil. Toss gently to combine.

7. Adjust the seasoning if needed. Serve the quinoa and roasted vegetable salad at room temperature or chilled. Enjoy!

Salmon and Avocado Salad with Lemon Vinaigrette

Ingredients:

- 2 salmon fillets

- Salt and pepper, to taste
- 4 cups mixed salad greens
- 1 avocado, sliced
- 1 cup cherry tomatoes, halved
- 1/4 cup sliced red onion
- Juice of 1 lemon
- 2 tablespoons extra-virgin olive oil
- 1 teaspoon Dijon mustard
- 1 teaspoon honey

Instructions:

1. Preheat the oven to 400°F (200°C).
2. Season the salmon fillets with salt and pepper. Place them on a baking sheet lined with parchment paper.
3. Bake the salmon in the preheated oven for 12-15 minutes, or until cooked through.
4. In a large bowl, combine the mixed salad greens, avocado slices, cherry tomatoes, and sliced red onion.
5. In a small bowl, whisk together the lemon juice, extra-virgin olive oil, Dijon mustard, honey, salt, and pepper to make the lemon vinaigrette.

6. Drizzle the lemon vinaigrette over the salad and toss
    gently to coat.

7. Divide the salad onto plates and top with the baked
    salmon fillets. Serve immediately and enjoy the
    refreshing flavors!

Chickpea and Vegetable Curry

Ingredients:

- 1 tablespoon coconut oil
- 1 onion, chopped
- 3 cloves garlic, minced
- 1 tablespoon grated fresh ginger
- 1 tablespoon curry powder
- 1 teaspoon ground turmeric
- 1 teaspoon ground cumin
- 1 can (14 ounces) chickpeas, drained and rinsed
- 1 can (14 ounces) diced tomatoes
- 1 cup coconut milk
- 2 cups chopped mixed vegetables (such as bell peppers, carrots, and zucchini)
- Salt and pepper, to taste

- Fresh cilantro, for garnish
- Cooked brown rice, for serving

Instructions:

1. Heat the coconut oil in a large pan over medium heat.
2. Add the chopped onion, minced garlic, and grated ginger to the pan. Sauté for 3-4 minutes, or until the onion becomes translucent.
3. Add the curry powder, ground turmeric, and ground cumin to the pan. Stir well to coat the onion mixture with the spices.
4. Add the chickpeas, diced tomatoes (with their juices), and coconut milk to the pan. Stir to combine.
5. Bring the mixture to a simmer and let it cook for 10 minutes, stirring occasionally.
6. Add the chopped mixed vegetables to the pan. Season with salt and pepper. Continue to simmer for another 10-15 minutes, or until the vegetables are tender.

7. Taste and adjust the seasoning if needed. Garnish with fresh cilantro.

8. Serve the chickpea and vegetable curry over cooked brown rice for a satisfying and flavorful lunch.

Turkey Lettuce Wraps with Hummus

Ingredients:

- 1 pound ground turkey
- 1 tablespoon olive oil
- 1 onion, finely chopped
- 2 cloves garlic, minced
- 1 teaspoon ground cumin
- 1 teaspoon ground coriander
- 1/2 teaspoon paprika
- Salt and pepper, to taste
- 8 large lettuce leaves (such as Bibb or romaine)
- 1/2 cup hummus
- 1/4 cup chopped fresh cilantro
- 1/4 cup diced tomatoes
- 1/4 cup diced cucumber
- 1/4 cup diced red bell pepper

Instructions:

1. Heat the olive oil in a large skillet over medium heat.
2. Add the chopped onion and minced garlic to the skillet. Sauté for 3-4 minutes, or until the onion becomes translucent.
3. Add the ground turkey to the skillet. Cook, breaking up the meat with a spoon, until it is browned and cooked through.
4. Stir in the ground cumin, ground coriander, paprika, salt, and pepper. Cook for an additional 2-3minutes to allow the flavors to meld.
5. Remove the skillet from heat. Drain any excess liquid if necessary.
6. Arrange the large lettuce leaves on a plate. Spread a spoonful of hummus onto each lettuce leaf.
7. Spoon the turkey mixture onto the lettuce leaves, dividing it evenly.
8. Top the turkey with chopped fresh cilantro, diced tomatoes, diced cucumber, and diced red bell pepper.

9. Roll up the lettuce leaves, securing them with toothpicks if desired.

10. Serve the turkey lettuce wraps as a light and refreshing lunch option. Enjoy the combination of flavors and textures!

Roasted Vegetable and Goat Cheese Tart

Ingredients:

- 1 sheet puff pastry, thawed
- 1 red bell pepper, thinly sliced
- 1 yellow bell pepper, thinly sliced
- 1 zucchini, thinly sliced
- 1 eggplant, thinly sliced
- 1 red onion, thinly sliced
- 2 tablespoons olive oil
- Salt and pepper, to taste
- 4 ounces goat cheese, crumbled
- Fresh basil leaves, for garnish

Instructions:

1. Preheat the oven to 400°F (200°C).

2. On a lightly floured surface, roll out the puff pastry sheet into a rectangle.

3. Transfer the rolled-out puff pastry onto a baking sheet lined with parchment paper.

4. In a large bowl, toss together the sliced red bell pepper, yellow bell pepper, zucchini, eggplant, and red onion with olive oil, salt, and pepper.

5. Spread the roasted vegetables evenly over the puff pastry, leaving a small border around the edges.

6. Crumble the goat cheese over the roasted vegetables.

7. Bake the tart in the preheated oven for 25-30 minutes, or until the puff pastry is golden brown and the vegetables are tender.

8. Remove the tart from the oven and let it cool slightly. Garnish with fresh basil leaves.

9. Slice the roasted vegetable and goat cheese tart into squares or wedges. Serve warm or at room temperature. Enjoy this delightful lunch option!

Asian Noodle Salad with Peanut Dressing

Ingredients:

- 8 ounces rice noodles
- 1 cup shredded carrots
- 1 cup shredded red cabbage
- 1/2 cup thinly sliced bell peppers
- 1/2 cup thinly sliced cucumbers
- 1/4 cup chopped scallions
- 1/4 cup chopped fresh cilantro
- 1/4 cup chopped roasted peanuts
- 2 tablespoons sesame seeds
- Lime wedges, for serving

For the Peanut Dressing:

- 1/4 cup creamy peanut butter
- 2 tablespoons soy sauce
- 2 tablespoons rice vinegar
- 1 tablespoon honey
- 1 tablespoon sesame oil
- 1 teaspoon grated fresh ginger
- 1 garlic clove, minced

- 2-3 tablespoons water (to thin the dressing)

Instructions:

1. Cook the rice noodles according to the package instructions. Drain and rinse with cold water to cool them down.
2. In a large bowl, combine the cooked rice noodles, shredded carrots, shredded red cabbage, thinly sliced bell peppers, thinly sliced cucumbers, chopped scallions, and chopped fresh cilantro.
3. In a small bowl, whisk together the creamy peanut butter, soy sauce, rice vinegar, honey, sesame oil, grated fresh ginger, and minced garlic to make the peanut dressing. Add water gradually to thin the dressing to your desired consistency.
4. Pour the peanut dressing over the noodle and vegetable mixture. Toss gently to coat everything in the dressing.
5. Sprinkle the chopped roasted peanuts and sesame seeds over the salad. Toss again to distribute the toppings evenly.

6. Serve the Asian noodle salad with lime wedges on the side. Squeeze fresh lime juice over the salad before enjoying its vibrant flavors.

Mediterranean Quinoa Stuffed Bell Peppers

Ingredients:

- 4 bell peppers (any color), tops removed and seeds removed
- 1 cup cooked quinoa
- 1 cup canned chickpeas, drained and rinsed
- 1/2 cup chopped sun-dried tomatoes
- 1/2 cup chopped Kalamata olives
- 1/4 cup crumbled feta cheese
- 2 tablespoons chopped fresh parsley
- 1 tablespoon lemon juice
- 1 tablespoon olive oil
- 2 teaspoons dried oregano
- Salt and pepper, to taste

Instructions:

1. Preheat the oven to 375°F (190°C).

2. Place the hollowed bell peppers in a baking dish, standing upright.

3. In a large bowl, combine the cooked quinoa, canned chickpeas, chopped sun-dried tomatoes, chopped Kalamata olives, crumbled feta cheese, chopped fresh parsley, lemon juice, olive oil, dried oregano, salt, and pepper. Mix well to combine all the ingredients.

4. Spoon the quinoa mixture into the bell peppers, pressing it down gently to fill them completely.

5. Cover the baking dish with foil and bake in the preheated oven for 25-30 minutes, or until the bell peppers are tender and the filling is heated through.

6. Remove the foil and continue to bake for an additional 5 minutes to allow the tops to brown slightly.

7. Carefully remove the stuffed bell peppers from the oven and let them cool for a few minutes before serving.

8. Serve the Mediterranean quinoa stuffed bell peppers as a wholesome and flavorful lunch. Enjoy the

delightful combination of Mediterranean ingredients!

Lentil Soup with Turmeric and Ginger

Ingredients:

- 1 tablespoon olive oil
- 1 onion, chopped
- 3 cloves garlic, minced
- 1 tablespoon grated fresh ginger
- 1 teaspoon ground turmeric
- 1/2 teaspoon ground cumin
- 1 cup dried lentils, rinsed and drained
- 4 cups vegetable broth
- 2 cups water
- 1 carrot, diced
- 1 celery stalk, diced
- 1 bay leaf
- Salt and pepper, to taste
- Fresh parsley, for garnish

Instructions:

1. Heat the olive oil in a large pot over medium heat.
2. Add the chopped onion, minced garlic, and grated ginger to the pot. Sauté for 3-4 minutes, or until the onion becomes translucent.
3. Stir in the ground turmeric and ground cumin. Cook for an additional minute to toast the spices.
4. Add the rinsed and drained lentils, vegetable broth, water, diced carrot, diced celery, bay leaf, salt, and pepper to the pot. Stir well to combine all the ingredients.
5. Bring the soup to a boil, then reduce heat to low. Cover the pot and let the soup simmer for 30-40 minutes, or until the lentils are tender.
6. Remove the bay leaf from the soup. Taste and adjust the seasoning if needed.
7. Ladle the lentil soup into bowls and garnish with fresh parsley.
8. Serve the comforting lentil soup with turmeric and ginger as a nourishing and filling lunch option.

Caprese Quinoa Salad with Balsamic Glaze

Ingredients:

- 1 cup cooked quinoa
- 1 cup cherry tomatoes, halved
- 1 cup fresh mozzarella pearls
- 1/2 cupchopped fresh basil leaves
- 2 tablespoons extra-virgin olive oil
- 1 tablespoon balsamic glaze
- Salt and pepper, to taste

Instructions:

1. In a large bowl, combine the cooked quinoa, cherry tomatoes, fresh mozzarella pearls, and chopped fresh basil.
2. Drizzle the extra-virgin olive oil and balsamic glaze over the salad.
3. Season with salt and pepper, then toss gently to coat all the ingredients.
4. Let the Caprese quinoa salad sit for a few minutes to allow the flavors to meld together.

5. Serve the salad at room temperature or chilled as a refreshing and nutritious lunch option. Enjoy the classic Caprese combination with a quinoa twist!

Chicken and Vegetable Stir-Fry

Ingredients:

- 2 boneless, skinless chicken breasts, thinly sliced
- 2 tablespoons soy sauce
- 1 tablespoon cornstarch
- 2 tablespoons sesame oil, divided
- 1 onion, sliced
- 2 cloves garlic, minced
- 1 bell pepper, sliced
- 1 cup broccoli florets
- 1 carrot, julienned
- 1 cup snap peas
- Salt and pepper, to taste
- Cooked brown rice, for serving

Instructions:

1. In a bowl, combine the thinly sliced chicken breasts with soy sauce and cornstarch. Toss to coat the chicken evenly and set aside.
2. Heat 1 tablespoon of sesame oil in a large skillet or wok over medium-high heat.
3. Add the sliced onion and minced garlic to the skillet. Stir-fry for 2-3 minutes, or until the onion becomes translucent.
4. Add the chicken to the skillet and stir-fry until it is cooked through and lightly browned. Remove the chicken from the skillet and set it aside.
5. In the same skillet, heat the remaining tablespoon of sesame oil.
6. Add the sliced bell pepper, broccoli florets, julienned carrot, and snap peas to the skillet. Stir-fry for 3-4 minutes, or until the vegetables are crisp-tender.
7. Return the cooked chicken to the skillet and stir to combine with the vegetables. Season with salt and pepper to taste.
8. Serve the chicken and vegetable stir-fry over cooked brown rice for a satisfying and wholesome

lunch. Enjoy the flavorful combination of tender chicken and crunchy vegetables!

Chapter 4: Dinner Recipes

In this chapter, we will explore a variety of delicious and nutritious dinner recipes that are designed to be both satisfying and anti-inflammatory. These recipes incorporate wholesome ingredients and vibrant flavors to create meals that not only support your overall health but also excite your taste buds. Let's dive into these mouthwatering dinner options:

Baked Salmon with Dill and Lemon

Ingredients:

- 4 salmon fillets
- 2 tablespoons fresh dill, chopped
- 1 lemon, sliced
- 2 tablespoons olive oil
- Salt and pepper to taste

Instructions:

1. Preheat the oven to 375°F (190°C).

2. Place the salmon fillets on a baking sheet lined with parchment paper.
3. Drizzle the olive oil over the salmon and season with salt and pepper.
4. Sprinkle the chopped dill evenly over the fillets.
5. Place a couple of lemon slices on top of each fillet.
6. Bake in the preheated oven for about 15-20 minutes, or until the salmon is cooked through and flakes easily with a fork.
7. Serve hot with your choice of roasted vegetables or a side salad.

Grilled Chicken Breast with Roasted Vegetables

Ingredients:

- 4 boneless, skinless chicken breasts
- 2 tablespoons olive oil
- 1 teaspoon dried herbs (such as thyme, rosemary, or Italian seasoning)
- Salt and pepper to taste

- Assorted vegetables for roasting (e.g., bell peppers, zucchini, onions, cherry tomatoes)

Instructions:

1. Preheat the grill to medium-high heat.
2. Season the chicken breasts with salt, pepper, and dried herbs.
3. Drizzle the chicken breasts with olive oil and rub the seasonings evenly.
4. Place the chicken breasts on the grill and cook for about 6-8 minutes per side, or until the internal temperature reaches 165°F (74°C).
5. While the chicken is grilling, prepare the roasted vegetables. Cut the vegetables into bite-sized pieces and toss them with olive oil, salt, and pepper.
6. Spread the vegetables on a baking sheet and roast in a preheated oven at 400°F (200°C) for about 15-20 minutes, or until they are tender and slightly caramelized.
7. Remove the chicken breasts from the grill and let them rest for a few minutes before serving.

8. Serve the grilled chicken breasts with a generous portion of roasted vegetables.

Quinoa and Black Bean Stuffed Peppers

Ingredients:

- 4 bell peppers (any color)
- 1 cup cooked quinoa
- 1 cup black beans, rinsed and drained
- 1/2 cup corn kernels (fresh or frozen)
- 1/2 cup diced tomatoes
- 1/4 cup diced red onion
- 1/4 cup chopped fresh cilantro
- 1 tablespoon lime juice
- 1 teaspoon ground cumin
- 1/2 teaspoon chili powder
- Salt and pepper to taste
- Shredded cheese for topping (optional)

Instructions:

1. Preheat the oven to 375°F (190°C).

2. Cut off the tops of the bell peppers and remove the seeds and membranes.
3. In a large bowl, combine the cooked quinoa, black beans, corn, diced tomatoes, red onion, cilantro, lime juice, cumin, chili powder, salt, and pepper. Mix well.
4. Stuff each bell pepper with the quinoa and black bean mixture, pressing it down gently.
5. Place the stuffed bell peppers in a baking dish and cover with aluminum foil.
6. Bake in the preheated oven for about 30-35 minutes, or until the peppers are tender and the filling is heated through.
7. If desired, remove the foil, sprinkle shredded cheese on top of each pepper, and return to the oven for an additional 5 minutes, or until the cheese is melted and bubbly.
8. Serve the stuffed peppers hot as a satisfying and flavorful dinner option.

Mediterranean Grilled Shrimp Skewers

Ingredients:

- 1 pound large shrimp, peeled and deveined
- 2 tablespoons olive oil
- 2 cloves garlic, minced
- 1 teaspoon dried oregano
- 1 teaspoon dried basil
- 1/2 teaspoon dried thyme
- Juice of 1 lemon
- Salt and pepper to taste
- Lemon wedges for serving

Instructions:

1. Preheat the grill to medium heat.
2. In a bowl, combine the olive oil, minced garlic, dried oregano, dried basil, dried thyme, lemon juice, salt, and pepper. Mix well.
3. Thread the shrimp onto skewers, piercing each shrimp near the tail and near the head to prevent it from curling.

4. Brush the shrimp skewers with the marinade, ensuring they are evenly coated.

5. Place the skewers on the preheated grill and cook for about 2-3 minutes per side, or until the shrimp turn pink and are cooked through.

6. Remove the shrimp skewers from the grill and squeeze fresh lemon juice over them.

7. Serve the Mediterranean grilled shrimp skewers with a side of your choice, such as a Greek salad or roasted vegetables.

Sweet Potato and Kale Curry

Ingredients:

- 2 large sweet potatoes, peeled and cubed
- 2 tablespoons coconut oil
- 1 onion, finely chopped
- 2 cloves garlic, minced
- 1 tablespoon grated fresh ginger
- 1 teaspoon ground turmeric
- 1 teaspoon ground cumin
- 1/2 teaspoon ground coriander

- 1/2 teaspoon paprika

- 1/4 teaspoon cayenne pepper (optional, for heat)

- 1 can (14 ounces) coconut milk

- 2 cups chopped kale

- Salt and pepper to taste

- Fresh cilantro for garnish

Instructions:

1. In a large skillet or pot, heat the coconut oil over medium heat.

2. Add the chopped onion, minced garlic, and grated ginger to the skillet. Sauté for about 3-4 minutes, or until the onion is translucent and fragrant.

3. Stir in the ground turmeric, ground cumin, ground coriander, paprika, and cayenne pepper (if using). Cook for another minute to toast the spices.

4. Add the cubed sweet potatoes to the skillet and toss them with the spice mixture until they are coated.

5. Pour in the coconut milk and bring the mixture to a simmer. Cover and cook for about 15-20 minutes, or until the sweet potatoes are tender.

6. Stir in the chopped kale and cook for an additional 5 minutes, or until the kale wilts.

7. Season the curry with salt and pepper to taste.

8. Serve the sweet potato and kale curry hot, garnished with fresh cilantro. It pairs well with steamed rice or naan bread.

Herb-Roasted Turkey Breast with Green Beans

Ingredients:

- 1 turkey breast (about 2-3 pounds)
- 2 tablespoons olive oil
- 2 cloves garlic, minced
- 1 tablespoon chopped fresh rosemary
- 1 tablespoon chopped fresh thyme
- Salt and pepper to taste
- 1 pound green beans, trimmed
- Lemon wedges for serving

Instructions:

1. Preheat the oven to 375°F (190°C).

2. Place the turkey breast in a roasting pan or baking
   dish.

3. In a small bowl, mix together the olive oil, minced
   garlic, chopped rosemary, chopped thyme, salt, and
   pepper.

4. Rub the herb mixture evenly over the turkey breast,
   ensuring it is well coated.

5. Arrange the green beans around the turkey breast in
   the roasting pan.

6. Roast in the preheated oven for about 60-70
   minutes, or until the turkey breast reaches an
   internal temperature of 165°F (74°C) and the juices
   run clear.

7. Remove the turkey breast from the oven and let it
   rest for a few minutes before slicing.

8. Serve the herb-roasted turkey breast with a side of
   roasted green beans and lemon wedges for an extra
   burst of freshness.

Lentil and Vegetable Casserole

Ingredients:

- 1 cup dried green or brown lentils
- 2 tablespoons olive oil
- 1 onion, chopped
- 2 carrots, diced
- 2 celery stalks, diced
- 2 cloves garlic, minced
- 1 teaspoon ground cumin
- 1 teaspoon ground coriander
- 1/2 teaspoon smoked paprika
- 1 can (14 ounces) diced tomatoes
- 2 cups vegetable broth
- Salt and pepper to taste
- 1/4 cup chopped fresh parsley for garnish

Instructions:

1. Rinse the lentils under cold water and drain.
2. In a large pot, heat the olive oil over medium heat.
3. Add the chopped onion, diced carrots, diced celery, and minced garlic to the pot. Sauté for about 5 minutes, or until the vegetables are softened.

4. Stir in the ground cumin, ground coriander, and smoked paprika. Cook for another minute to toast the spices.

5. Add the rinsed lentils, diced tomatoes, and vegetable broth to the pot. Bring the mixture to a boil, then reduce the heat to low.

6. Cover the pot and simmer for about 30-40 minutes, or until the lentils are tender and most of the liquid is absorbed.

7. Season the lentil and vegetable casserole with salt and pepper to taste.

8. Serve the casserole hot, garnished with chopped fresh parsley. It makes a satisfying and nutritious dinner option on its own or paired with a side salad.

Spaghetti Squash with Tomato Basil Sauce

Ingredients:

- 1 spaghetti squash
- 2 tablespoons olive oil
- 1 onion, chopped

- 2 cloves garlic, minced
- 1 can (14 ounces) diced tomatoes
- 1/4 cup tomato paste
- 1/4 cup chopped fresh basil
- 1 teaspoon dried oregano
- Salt and pepper to taste
- Grated Parmesan cheese for serving (optional)

Instructions:

1. Preheat the oven to 400°F (200°C).
2. Cut the spaghetti squash in half lengthwise and scoop out the seeds.
3. Place the squash halves cut side down on a baking sheet lined with parchment paper.
4. Bake in the preheated oven for about 40-50 minutes, or until the squash is tender and the strands easily separate with a fork.
5. While the squash is baking, prepare the tomato basil sauce. In a saucepan, heat the olive oil over medium heat.

6. Add the chopped onion and minced garlic to the saucepan. Sauté for about 5 minutes, or until the onion is translucent and fragrant.

7. Stir in the diced tomatoes, tomato paste, chopped basil, dried oregano, salt, and pepper. Simmer for about 15-20 minutes, allowing the flavors to meld together.

8. Once the spaghetti squash is cooked, use a fork to scrape the flesh into strands, resembling spaghetti.

9. Serve the spaghetti squash with a generous ladle of tomato basil sauce on top. Sprinkle with grated Parmesan cheese, if desired, for an added touch of flavor.

Ginger and Garlic Glazed Tofu with Stir-Fried Vegetables

Ingredients:

- 1 block (14 ounces) firm tofu, drained and cut into cubes
- 2 tablespoons soy sauce
- 1 tablespoon sesame oil

- 2 cloves garlic, minced
- 1 tablespoon grated fresh ginger
- 2 tablespoons honey or maple syrup
- 2 tablespoons rice vinegar
- 2 tablespoons vegetable oil
- Assorted vegetables for stir-frying (e.g., bell peppers, broccoli, carrots, snap peas)
- Cooked brown rice for serving

Instructions:

1. In a bowl, whisk together the soy sauce, sesame oil, minced garlic, grated ginger, honey or maple syrup, and rice vinegar.
2. Place the tofu cubes in the marinade and gently toss to coat. Let it marinate for at least 15 minutes, allowing the flavors to penetrate the tofu.
3. Heat the vegetable oil in a large skillet or wok over medium-high heat.
4. Remove the tofu cubes from the marinade, reserving the marinade for later use.
5. Add the tofu to the skillet and cook for about 5-7 minutes, or until golden and slightly crispy on the

outside. Turn the tofu cubes occasionally to ensure even cooking.

6. Remove the tofu from the skillet and set it aside.
7. In the same skillet, add the assorted vegetables for stir-frying. Cook for about 5-7 minutes, or until the vegetables are crisp-tender.
8. Pour the reserved marinade into the skillet and cook for an additional 2-3 minutes, allowing the sauce to thicken slightly.
9. Return the cooked tofu to the skillet and toss it with the stir-fried vegetables and sauce.
10. Serve the ginger and garlic glazed tofu with stir-fried vegetables over a bed of cooked brown rice for a flavorful and satisfying dinner option.

Beef and Broccoli Stir-Fry

Ingredients:

- 1 pound beef sirloin or flank steak, thinly sliced
- 1/4 cup low-sodium soy sauce
- 2 tablespoons oyster sauce
- 1 tablespoon cornstarch

- 2 tablespoons vegetable oil
- 3 cloves garlic, minced
- 1 tablespoon grated fresh ginger
- 2 cups broccoli florets
- 1 cup sliced bell peppers
- 1/2 cup sliced mushrooms
- Salt and pepper to taste
- Cooked rice or noodles for serving

Instructions:

1. In a bowl, whisk together the soy sauce, oyster sauce, and cornstarch. Set aside.
2. Heat the vegetable oil in a large skillet or wok over high heat.
3. Add the minced garlic and grated ginger to the skillet. Stir-fry for about 1 minute, or until fragrant.
4. Add the thinly sliced beef to the skillet and cook for about 2-3 minutes, or untilthe beef is browned and cooked through. Remove the beef from the skillet and set it aside.
5. In the same skillet, add the broccoli florets, sliced bell peppers, and sliced mushrooms. Stir-fry for

about 3-4 minutes, or until the vegetables are crisp-tender.

6. Return the cooked beef to the skillet and pour the sauce mixture over the beef and vegetables.

7. Stir-fry for an additional 2-3 minutes, or until the sauce thickens and coats the beef and vegetables evenly.

8. Season with salt and pepper to taste.

9. Serve the beef and broccoli stir-fry hot over cooked rice or noodles for a delicious and satisfying dinner option.

Eggplant Parmesan with Marinara Sauce

Ingredients:

- 2 large eggplants
- Salt for sprinkling
- 2 cups breadcrumbs
- 1 cup grated Parmesan cheese
- 2 teaspoons dried Italian seasoning
- 2 eggs, beaten

- 1/4 cup olive oil

- 2 cups marinara sauce

- 1 cup shredded mozzarella cheese

- Fresh basil leaves for garnish

Instructions:

1. Preheat the oven to 375°F (190°C).

2. Slice the eggplants into rounds, about 1/4 inch thick. Place the eggplant slices on a baking sheet lined with parchment paper.

3. Sprinkle salt over the eggplant slices and let them sit for about 20 minutes. This helps draw out any excess moisture and bitterness from the eggplants.

4. In a shallow dish, combine the breadcrumbs, grated Parmesan cheese, and dried Italian seasoning.

5. Dip each eggplant slice into the beaten eggs, then coat it in the breadcrumb mixture, pressing gently to adhere.

6. Heat the olive oil in a large skillet over medium heat. Working in batches, cook the breaded eggplant slices for about 2-3 minutes per side, or until golden brown. Place the cooked eggplant

slices on a paper towel-lined plate to absorb any excess oil.

7. In a baking dish, spread a thin layer of marinara sauce on the bottom.

8. Arrange a layer of cooked eggplant slices on top of the marinara sauce. Repeat the process, alternating layers of eggplant and marinara sauce until all the eggplant slices are used.

9. Pour the remaining marinara sauce over the top layer of eggplant.

10. Sprinkle the shredded mozzarella cheese over the sauce.

11. Bake in the preheated oven for about 25-30 minutes, or until the cheese is melted and bubbly.

12. Remove the eggplant Parmesan from the oven and let it rest for a few minutes.

13. Garnish with fresh basil leaves before serving. This classic Italian dish is perfect for a comforting and flavorful dinner.

Chapter 5: Snacks and Appetizers

Enjoy these delicious and healthy snacks and appetizers from Chapter 5 of the "28-Day Prevention Anti-Inflammatory Cookbook"!

Roasted Red Pepper Hummus with Crudites

Ingredients:

- 1 can (15 ounces) chickpeas, drained and rinsed
- 1 roasted red pepper, drained
- 2 tablespoons tahini
- 2 tablespoons lemon juice
- 2 cloves garlic, minced
- 2 tablespoons olive oil
- 1/2 teaspoon cumin
- Salt and pepper to taste
- Assorted fresh vegetables (crudites) for serving (carrots, celery, bell peppers, etc.)

Instructions:

1. In a food processor, combine the chickpeas, roasted red pepper, tahini, lemon juice, minced garlic, olive oil, cumin, salt, and pepper.
2. Process until smooth and creamy, scraping down the sides as needed.
3. Taste and adjust the seasonings if necessary.
4. Transfer the hummus to a serving bowl and refrigerate for at least 1 hour to allow the flavors to meld.
5. Serve with an assortment of fresh vegetables for dipping.

Greek Yogurt and Cucumber Dip

Ingredients:

- 1 cup Greek yogurt
- 1/2 cucumber, grated and squeezed to remove excess moisture
- 2 cloves garlic, minced
- 1 tablespoon lemon juice
- 1 tablespoon fresh dill, chopped
- Salt and pepper to taste
- Pita bread or chips for serving

Instructions:

1. In a bowl, combine the Greek yogurt, grated cucumber, minced garlic, lemon juice, chopped dill, salt, and pepper.
2. Stir well to combine all the ingredients.
3. Taste and adjust the seasonings if needed.
4. Cover the bowl and refrigerate for at least 30 minutes to allow the flavors to develop.
5. Serve the dip chilled with pita bread or chips.

Baked Kale Chips with Sea Salt

Ingredients:

- 1 bunch kale, washed and dried
- 1 tablespoon olive oil
- Sea salt to taste

Instructions:

1. Preheat your oven to 350°F (175°C) and line a baking sheet with parchment paper.
2. Remove the tough stems from the kale leaves and tear the leaves into bite-sized pieces.

3. In a large bowl, drizzle the kale leaves with olive oil and sprinkle with sea salt.

4. Toss the leaves gently to evenly coat them with oil and salt.

5. Spread the kale leaves in a single layer on the prepared baking sheet.

6. Bake for 10-15 minutes, or until the leaves are crispy and slightly golden.

7. Remove from the oven and let the kale chips cool completely before serving.

Smoked Salmon Roll-Ups with Cream Cheese

Ingredients:

- 4 ounces smoked salmon
- 4 ounces cream cheese
- 1 tablespoon fresh dill, chopped
- 1 tablespoon capers (optional)
- Freshly ground black pepper
- Lemon wedges for serving

Instructions:

1. Lay the smoked salmon slices flat on a cutting
   board.
2. In a small bowl, mix together the cream cheese,
   chopped dill, capers (if using), and a pinch of
   freshly ground black pepper.
3. Spread a thin layer of the cream cheese mixture
   evenly onto each smoked salmon slice.
4. Roll up the smoked salmon tightly, starting from
   one end.
5. Slice the rolled-up salmon into bite-sized pieces.
6. Serve the smoked salmon roll-ups with lemon
   wedges on the side.

Caprese Skewers with Balsamic Glaze

Ingredients:

- Cherry tomatoes
- Fresh mozzarella balls (ciliegine)
- Fresh basil leaves
- Balsamic glaze

Instructions:

1. Assemble the skewers by threading one cherry tomato, one mozzarella ball, and one basil leaf onto each skewer.

2. Repeat until all the ingredients are used.

3. Place the skewers on a serving platter.

4. Drizzle the caprese skewers with balsamic glaze just before serving.

5. Serve immediately.

Zucchini Fritters with Yogurt Sauce

Ingredients:

- 2 medium zucchini, grated
- 1/2 teaspoon salt
- 1/4 cup all-purpose flour
- 1/4 cup grated Parmesan cheese
- 2 green onions, thinly sliced
- 1 large egg, beaten
- 2 tablespoons chopped fresh parsley
- 1/4 teaspoon black pepper
- 2 tablespoons olive oil (for frying)
- Greek yogurt sauce for serving (see instructions below)

Instructions:

1. Place the grated zucchini in a colander and sprinkle with salt.
2. Let it sit for about 10 minutes to allow the excess moisture to drain.
3. After 10 minutes, squeeze the zucchini to remove as much liquid as possible.
4. In a mixing bowl, combine the drained zucchini, flour, grated Parmesan cheese, sliced green onions, beaten egg, chopped parsley, and black pepper.
5. Stir until all the ingredients are well combined.
6. Heat the olive oil in a large skillet over medium heat.
7. Drop spoonfuls of the zucchini mixture into the skillet, flattening them slightly with the back of the spoon.
8. Cook the fritters for 2-3 minutes on each side, or until they turn golden brown.
9. Remove the fritters from the skillet and drain them on a paper towel-lined plate.
10. Repeat the process with the remaining zucchini mixture, adding more oil if necessary.

11. For the yogurt sauce, simply mix Greek yogurt with a pinch of salt and pepper.

12. Serve the zucchini fritters warm with the yogurt sauce.

Spicy Roasted Chickpeas

Ingredients:

- 1 can (15 ounces) chickpeas, drained and rinsed
- 2 tablespoons olive oil
- 1 teaspoon ground cumin
- 1 teaspoon chili powder
- 1/2 teaspoon garlic powder
- 1/2 teaspoon paprika
- 1/4 teaspoon cayenne pepper (adjust to taste)
- Salt to taste

Instructions:

1. Preheat your oven to 400°F (200°C) and line a baking sheet with parchment paper.

2. Pat the chickpeas dry with a paper towel to remove excess moisture.

3. In a bowl, toss the chickpeas with olive oil, cumin, chili powder, garlic powder, paprika, cayenne pepper, and salt.
4. Spread the seasoned chickpeas in a single layer on the prepared baking sheet.
5. Roast in the preheated oven for 20-25 minutes, or until the chickpeas are crispy and golden.
6. Remove from the oven and let them cool slightly before serving.

Guacamole with Baked Tortilla Chips

Ingredients:

- 2 ripe avocados
- 1 small tomato, diced
- 1/4 cup red onion, finely chopped
- 1 jalapeno pepper, seeded and minced
- 2 tablespoons fresh cilantro, chopped
- 1 tablespoon lime juice
- 1/2 teaspoon cumin
- Salt and pepper to taste
- Baked tortilla chips for serving

Instructions:

1. Cut the avocados in half, remove the pits, and scoop the flesh intoa bowl.
2. Mash the avocados with a fork until desired consistency.
3. Add the diced tomato, chopped red onion, minced jalapeno pepper, chopped cilantro, lime juice, cumin, salt, and pepper.
4. Mix well until all the ingredients are combined.
5. Taste and adjust the seasonings if needed.
6. Cover the bowl with plastic wrap, making sure it touches the surface of the guacamole to prevent browning.
7. Refrigerate for at least 30 minutes to allow the flavors to meld.
8. Serve the guacamole with baked tortilla chips.

Stuffed Mushrooms with Spinach and Feta

Ingredients:

- 12 large mushrooms, stems removed
- 1 tablespoon olive oil

- 2 cloves garlic, minced
- 2 cups fresh spinach, chopped
- 1/4 cup crumbled feta cheese
- Salt and pepper to taste

Instructions:

1. Preheat your oven to 375°F (190°C) and line a baking sheet with parchment paper.
2. Place the mushroom caps on the prepared baking sheet, gill-side up.
3. In a skillet, heat the olive oil over medium heat.
4. Add the minced garlic and sauté for 1 minute until fragrant.
5. Add the chopped spinach to the skillet and cook until wilted, about 2-3 minutes.
6. Remove the skillet from heat and let the spinach cool slightly.
7. Once the spinach has cooled, stir in the crumbled feta cheese, salt, and pepper.
8. Spoon the spinach and feta mixture into the mushroom caps, filling them generously.

9. Bake the stuffed mushrooms in the preheated oven for 15-20 minutes, or until the mushrooms are tender and the filling is lightly browned.

10. Remove from the oven and let them cool for a few minutes before serving.

Buffalo Cauliflower Bites

Ingredients:

- 1 head cauliflower, cut into bite-sized florets
- 1/2 cup all-purpose flour
- 1/2 cup milk (dairy or plant-based)
- 1/2 teaspoon garlic powder
- 1/2 teaspoon onion powder
- 1/4 teaspoon paprika
- 1/4 teaspoon salt
- 1/4 teaspoon black pepper
- 1/4 cup hot sauce
- 2 tablespoons melted butter (or olive oil for a dairy-free option)
- Ranch or blue cheese dressing for dipping (optional)

Instructions:

1. Preheat your oven to 450°F (230°C) and line a baking sheet with parchment paper.
2. In a large bowl, whisk together the flour, milk, garlic powder, onion powder, paprika, salt, and black pepper until smooth.
3. Add the cauliflower florets to the bowl and toss to coat them evenly with the batter.
4. Arrange the coated cauliflower florets in a single layer on the prepared baking sheet.
5. Bake for 20-25 minutes, or until the cauliflower is golden brown and crispy.
6. In a separate bowl, whisk together the hot sauce and melted butter.
7. Once the cauliflower is done baking, remove it from the oven and drizzle the hot sauce mixture over the florets.
8. Toss the cauliflower gently to coat it evenly with the buffalo sauce.
9. Return the baking sheet to the oven and bake for an additional 5 minutes to allow the sauce to soak into the cauliflower.

10. Remove from the oven and let the buffalo cauliflower bites cool slightly before serving.

11. Serve with ranch or blue cheese dressing for dipping, if desired.

Quinoa and Spinach Bites

Ingredients:

- 1 cup cooked quinoa
- 1 cup fresh spinach, chopped
- 1/4 cup grated Parmesan cheese
- 1/4 cup shredded mozzarella cheese
- 2 green onions, thinly sliced
- 1 clove garlic, minced
- 1/2 teaspoon dried oregano
- 1/4 teaspoon salt
- 1/4 teaspoon black pepper
- 2 large eggs, beaten

Instructions:

1. Preheat your oven to 350°F (175°C) and line a baking sheet with parchment paper.

2. In a large bowl, combine the cooked quinoa, chopped spinach, grated Parmesan cheese, shredded mozzarella cheese, sliced green onions, minced garlic, dried oregano, salt, black pepper, and beaten eggs.
3. Stir well until all the ingredients are thoroughly combined.
4. Scoop about 1 tablespoon of the quinoa mixture and shape it into a bite-sized ball using your hands.
5. Place the quinoa ball onto the prepared baking sheet.
6. Repeat the process with the remaining quinoa mixture, spacing the balls about 1 inch apart.
7. Bake in the preheated oven for 15-20 minutes, or until the quinoa bites are golden brown and firm to the touch.
8. Remove from the oven and let them cool for a few minutes before serving.

In this chapter, you'll discover a delightful array of desserts that are not only delicious but also anti-inflammatory. These sweet treats are designed to satisfy your cravings while providing nourishment and promoting overall well-being. Indulge in these guilt-free desserts and let their flavors bring you joy and satisfaction.

Mixed Berry Parfait with Greek Yogurt

Ingredients:

- 1 cup mixed berries (strawberries, blueberries, raspberries)
- 1 cup Greek yogurt
- 1 tablespoon honey or maple syrup
- 1/4 cup granola

Instructions:

1. Wash the mixed berries and pat them dry. Slice the strawberries into bite-sized pieces.

2. In a glass or a bowl, layer the Greek yogurt, mixed
    berries, and granola.

3. Drizzle honey or maple syrup over the top for added
    sweetness.

4. Repeat the layers until all the ingredients are used,
    finishing with a layer of berries on top.

5. Serve chilled and enjoy this refreshing and
    nutritious parfait.

Dark Chocolate Avocado Mousse

Ingredients:

- 2 ripe avocados
- 1/4 cup unsweetened cocoa powder
- 1/4 cup maple syrup or honey
- 1/2 teaspoon vanilla extract
- Pinch of sea salt
- Fresh berries, for garnish

Instructions:

1. Cut the avocados in half, remove the pits, and scoop
    out the flesh.

2. In a blender or food processor, combine the avocado flesh, cocoa powder, maple syrup or honey, vanilla extract, and sea salt.

3. Blend until smooth and creamy, scraping down the sides if needed.

4. Spoon the chocolate avocado mousse into serving glasses or bowls.

5. Refrigerate for at least 1 hour to allow the mousse to set.

6. Garnish with fresh berries before serving. Indulge in this luscious and guilt-free chocolate treat.

Baked Apples with Cinnamon and Walnuts

Ingredients:

- 4 apples (Granny Smith or Honeycrisp)
- 1/4 cup chopped walnuts
- 2 tablespoons honey or maple syrup
- 1 teaspoon ground cinnamon
- 1/4 teaspoon nutmeg
- 2 tablespoons coconut oil, melted

Instructions:

1. Preheat the oven to 375°F (190°C). Line a baking dish with parchment paper.
2. Core the apples using an apple corer or a small knife, leaving the bottoms intact.
3. In a small bowl, mix the chopped walnuts, honey or maple syrup, cinnamon, and nutmeg.
4. Stuff each apple with the walnut mixture, dividing it evenly among them.
5. Place the stuffed apples in the prepared baking dish.
6. Drizzle melted coconut oil over the apples.
7. Bake for 25-30 minutes, or until the apples are tender.
8. Remove from the oven and let them cool slightly before serving. These baked apples make a comforting and aromatic dessert.

Coconut Chia Pudding with Mango

Ingredients:

- 1/4 cup chia seeds
- 1 cup coconut milk
- 1 tablespoon maple syrup or honey

- 1/2 teaspoon vanilla extract
- 1 ripe mango, diced
- Shredded coconut, for garnish

Instructions:

1. In a bowl, combine the chia seeds, coconut milk, maple syrup or honey, and vanilla extract.
2. Stir well to ensure the chia seeds are evenly distributed.
3. Let the mixture sit for 10 minutes, then stir again to break up any clumps.
4. Cover the bowl and refrigerate overnight or for at least 4 hours, allowing the chia seeds to absorb the liquid and create a pudding-like consistency.
5. In serving glasses or bowls, layer the coconut chia pudding and diced mango.
6. Garnish with shredded coconut before serving. Enjoy this tropical and creamy chia pudding!

Almond Flour Blueberry Muffins

Ingredients:

- 2 cups almond flour

- 1/4 cup coconut flour
- 1 teaspoon baking soda
- 1/4 teaspoon salt
- 3 eggs
- 1/4 cup maple syrup or honey
- 1/4 cup coconut oil, melted
- 1 teaspoon vanilla extract
- 1 cup blueberries

Instructions:

1. Preheat the oven to 350°F (175°C). Line a muffin tin with paper liners.
2. In a large bowl, whisk together the almond flour, coconut flour, baking soda, and salt.
3. In a separate bowl, whisk together the eggs, maple syrup or honey, melted coconut oil, and vanilla extract.
4. Pour the wet ingredients into the dry ingredients and stir until well combined.
5. Gently fold in the blueberries.
6. Spoon the batter into the prepared muffin tin, filling each cup about three-quarters full.

7. Bake for 20-25 minutes, or until a toothpick inserted into the center of a muffin comes out clean.

8. Allow the muffins to cool for a few minutes before transferring them to a wire rack to cool completely. These almond flour blueberry muffins are a delightful and nutritious treat.

Banana Ice Cream with Almond Butter Swirl

Ingredients:

- 4 ripe bananas, peeled and frozen
- 2 tablespoons almond butter
- 2 tablespoons chopped dark chocolate (optional)

Instructions:

1. Place the frozen bananas in a blender or food processor.

2. Blend until smooth and creamy, scraping down the sides as needed.

3. Add the almond butter and blend again until well combined.

4. If desired, fold in the chopped dark chocolate for added texture and flavor.

5. Transfer the banana ice cream to a freezer-safe container and freeze for 1-2 hours to firm up.

6. Scoop into bowls or cones and enjoy this guilt-free and creamy banana ice cream with a delicious almond butter swirl.

Lemon Poppy Seed Energy Balls

Ingredients:

- 1 cup dates, pitted
- 1 cup raw cashews
- 1/4 cup unsweetened shredded coconut
- Zest and juice of 1 lemon
- 2 tablespoons poppy seeds

Instructions:

1. Place the dates, cashews, shredded coconut, lemon zest, and lemon juice in a food processor.

2. Process until the ingredients are well combined and form a sticky dough.

3. Add the poppy seeds and pulse a few times to incorporate them into the mixture.

4. Using your hands, roll the mixture into bite-sized balls.

5. Place the energy balls on a baking sheet lined with parchment paper.

6. Refrigerate for at least 1 hour to allow them to firm up.

7. Store in an airtight container in the refrigerator for up to one week. These lemon poppy seed energy balls are perfect for a quick and energizing snack.

Raspberry Coconut Bars

Ingredients:

- 1 cup almonds
- 1 cup unsweetened shredded coconut
- 1/4 cup coconut oil, melted
- 2 tablespoons maple syrup or honey
- 1 cup fresh raspberries

Instructions:

1. Preheat the oven to 350°F (175°C). Line an 8x8-inch baking dish with parchment paper.
2. In a food processor, pulse the almonds until finely ground.
3. Add the shredded coconut, melted coconut oil, and maple syrup or honey to the food processor.
4. Process until the mixture comes together and forms a sticky crust.
5. Press the crust mixture evenly into the bottom of the prepared baking dish.
6. Bake for 10-12 minutes, or until the crust is golden brown.
7. Remove from the oven and let it cool completely.
8. Spread the fresh raspberries evenly over the cooled crust.
9. Place the dish in the refrigerator for at least 1 hour to allow the bars to set.
10. Once set, cut into squares and serve these delightful raspberry coconut bars.

Pumpkin Pie Chia Pudding

Ingredients:

- 1/4 cup chia seeds
- 1 cup unsweetened almond milk
- 1/4 cup pumpkin puree
- 2 tablespoons maple syrup or honey
- 1/2 teaspoon pumpkin pie spice
- Pecans or walnuts, for topping

Instructions:

1. In a bowl, combine the chia seeds, almond milk, pumpkin puree, maple syrup or honey, and pumpkin pie spice.
2. Stir well to ensure the chia seeds are evenly distributed and there are no clumps.
3. Let the mixture sit for 10 minutes, then stir again.
4. Cover the bowl and refrigerate overnight or for at least 4 hours, allowing the chia seeds to absorb the liquid and create a pudding-like consistency.
5. Before serving, give the pudding a good stir to make it smooth and creamy.

6. Top with pecans or walnuts for added crunch and enjoy this seasonal pumpkin pie chia pudding.

Berry Crumble with Oat Topping

Ingredients:

- 4 cups mixed berries (strawberries, blueberries, raspberries)
- 1 tablespoon lemon juice
- 2 tablespoons maple syrup or honey
- 1 cup rolled oats
- 1/2 cup almond flour
- 1/4 cup coconut oil, melted
- 2 tablespoons maple syrup or honey
- 1/2 teaspoon cinnamon
- Pinch of salt

Instructions:

1. Preheat the oven to 375°F (190°C). Grease a baking dish with coconut oil or cooking spray.
2. In a bowl, combine the mixed berries, lemon juice, and maple syrup or honey. Toss gently to coat the berries.

3. Transfer the berry mixture to the prepared baking dish, spreading it evenly.

4. In another bowl, combine the rolled oats, almond flour, melted coconut oil, maple syrup or honey, cinnamon, and salt. Mix until the ingredients are well combined and crumbly.

5. Sprinkle the oat topping evenly over the berries in the baking dish.

6. Bake for 25-30 minutes, or until the topping is golden brown and the berries are bubbling.

7. Remove from the oven and let it cool for a few minutes before serving. Serve this warm and comforting berry crumble with a scoop of vanilla ice cream or a dollop of Greek yogurt.

Chocolate Peanut Butter Protein Balls

Ingredients:

- 1 cup rolled oats
- 1/2 cup chocolate protein powder
- 1/2 cup natural peanut butter
- 1/4 cup honey

- 2 tablespoons unsweetened cocoa powder
- 2 tablespoons unsweetened almond milk
- 1/4 cup dark chocolate chips (optional)

Instructions:

1. In a large bowl, combine the rolled oats, chocolate protein powder, peanut butter, honey, cocoa powder, and almond milk.
2. Stir well until all the ingredients are thoroughly combined and form a sticky mixture.
3. If desired, fold in the dark chocolate chips for added richness.
4. Using your hands, roll the mixture into bite-sized balls.
5. Place the protein balls on a baking sheet lined with parchment paper.
6. Refrigerate for at least 1 hour to allow them to firm up.
7. Store in an airtight container in the refrigerator for up to one week. These chocolate peanut butter protein balls make a nutritious and satisfying snack.

Green Detox Smoothie with Spinach and Pineapple

Ingredients:

- 1 cup fresh spinach leaves
- 1 cup chopped pineapple
- 1 medium banana
- ½ cup coconut water
- ½ cup almond milk
- 1 tablespoon chia seeds
- 1 tablespoon honey (optional)

Instructions:

1. In a blender, add the spinach leaves, chopped pineapple, banana, coconut water, almond milk, chia seeds, and honey (if desired).
2. Blend on high speed until smooth and creamy.
3. Pour into a glass and enjoy this refreshing and detoxifying green smoothie.

Berry Blast Smoothie with Almond Milk

Ingredients:

- 1 cup mixed berries (strawberries, blueberries, raspberries)
- 1 cup almond milk
- ½ cup Greek yogurt
- 1 tablespoon honey
- 1 tablespoon flaxseeds

Instructions:

1. Place the mixed berries, almond milk, Greek yogurt, honey, and flaxseeds in a blender.
2. Blend until the ingredients are well combined and the smoothie is thick and creamy.
3. Pour into a glass and savor the burst of berry flavors in this nutritious smoothie.

Mango Turmeric Smoothie with Coconut Water

Ingredients:

- 1 ripe mango, peeled and pitted
- ½ cup coconut water
- ½ cup plain yogurt
- 1 teaspoon turmeric powder
- 1 tablespoon honey (optional)
- Juice of 1 lime

Instructions:

1. Add the ripe mango, coconut water, plain yogurt, turmeric powder, honey (if desired), and lime juice to a blender.
2. Blend until the mixture is smooth and creamy.
3. Pour into a glass and enjoy the tropical goodness of this mango turmeric smoothie.

Chocolate Banana Protein Smoothie

Ingredients:

- 1 ripe banana

- 1 cup almond milk

- 2 tablespoons chocolate protein powder

- 1 tablespoon almond butter

- 1 tablespoon honey (optional)

- Ice cubes (optional)

Instructions:

1. Place the ripe banana, almond milk, chocolate protein powder, almond butter, honey (if desired), and ice cubes (if using) into a blender.

2. Blend until all the ingredients are well combined and the smoothie is creamy.

3. Pour into a glass and indulge in the rich and chocolatey goodness of this protein-packed smoothie.

Pineapple and Ginger Smoothie with Flaxseeds

Ingredients:

- 1 cup chopped pineapple

- 1-inch piece of fresh ginger, peeled

- ½ cup coconut water

- ½ cup Greek yogurt

- 1 tablespoon flaxseeds

- 1 tablespoon honey (optional)

- Juice of 1 lemon

Instructions:

1. Add the chopped pineapple, fresh ginger, coconut water, Greek yogurt, flaxseeds, honey (if desired), and lemon juice to a blender.

2. Blend until the ingredients are well combined and the smoothie is smooth and frothy.

3. Pour into a glass and enjoy the tropical flavors with a hint of ginger in this revitalizing smoothie.

Creamy Avocado and Spinach Smoothie

Ingredients:

- 1 ripe avocado, peeled and pitted

- 1 cup fresh spinach leaves

- 1 cup almond milk

- ½ cup Greek yogurt

- 1 tablespoon honey (optional)

- Juice of 1 lime

Instructions:

1. Place the ripe avocado, fresh spinach leaves, almond milk, Greek yogurt, honey (if desired), and lime juice into a blender.

2. Blend until the mixture is creamy and well blended.

3. Pour into a glass and savor the creamy texture and the nutritious combination of avocado and spinach in this smoothie.

Blueberry Almond Butter Smoothie

Ingredients:

- 1 cup blueberries

- 1 cup almond milk

- 2 tablespoons almond butter

- 1 tablespoon honey

- ½ teaspoon vanilla extract

Instructions:

1. In a blender, add the blueberries, almond milk, almond butter, honey, and vanilla extract.
2. Blend until the ingredients are smooth and well incorporated.
3. Pour into a glass and enjoy the delightful combination of blueberries and almond butter in this satisfying smoothie.

Tropical Mango Pineapple Smoothie

Ingredients:

- 1 cup chopped mango
- 1 cup chopped pineapple
- ½ cup coconut milk
- ½ cup orange juice
- 1 tablespoon shredded coconut (optional)
- Ice cubes (optional)

Instructions:

1. Add the chopped mango, chopped pineapple, coconut milk, orange juice, shredded coconut (if desired), and ice cubes (if using) to a blender.

2. Blend until all the ingredients are well combined and the smoothie is creamy and tropical.

3. Pour into a glass and transport yourself to a beachside paradise with this luscious mango pineapple smoothie.

Beet and Berry Smoothie with Greek Yogurt

Ingredients:

- 1 small beet, peeled and chopped
- 1 cup mixed berries (strawberries, blueberries, raspberries)
- ½ cup Greek yogurt
- 1 tablespoon honey
- 1 tablespoon chia seeds

Instructions:

1. Place the chopped beet, mixed berries, Greek yogurt, honey, and chia seeds in a blender.

2. Blend until the ingredients are smooth and the smoothie has a vibrant color.

3. Pour into a glass and enjoy the sweet and earthy flavors of this nutritious beet and berry smoothie.

Peanut Butter and Banana Smoothie

Ingredients:

- 1 ripe banana
- 2 tablespoons peanut butter
- 1 cup almond milk
- ½ cup Greek yogurt
- 1 tablespoon honey (optional)
- 1 tablespoon cocoa powder (optional)

Instructions:

1. Add the ripe banana, peanut butter, almond milk, Greek yogurt, honey (if desired), and cocoa powder (if using) to a blender.

2. Blend until all the ingredients are well combined
    and the smoothie is creamy and smooth.

3. Pour into a glass and relish the classic combination
    of peanut butter and banana in this delicious
    smoothie.

Orange Carrot Ginger Smoothie

Ingredients:

- 1 large carrot, peeled and chopped
- Juice of 2 oranges
- 1-inch piece of fresh ginger, peeled
- ½ cup coconut water
- 1 tablespoon honey (optional)
- Ice cubes (optional)

Instructions:

1. Place the chopped carrot, orange juice, fresh ginger,
    coconut water, honey (if desired), and ice cubes (if
    using) in a blender.

2. Blend until the ingredients are well combined and
    the smoothie is smooth and refreshing.

3. Pour into a glass and enjoy the zesty flavors of orange, carrot, and ginger in this invigorating smoothie.

CONCLUSION

As we conclude our 28-day journey, it is important to recognize that this is just the beginning. Incorporating the principles of an anti-inflammatory diet into our everyday lives is crucial for long-term success. To that end, here are some essential tips to help you maintain an anti-inflammatory lifestyle:

Emphasize whole foods: Make whole grains, fresh fruits and vegetables, lean proteins, and healthy fats the foundation of your meals. Minimize processed foods, refined sugars, and unhealthy fats, as they can trigger inflammation.

Experiment with herbs and spices: Utilize the power of herbs and spices to enhance the flavor of your dishes. Turmeric, ginger, cinnamon, and garlic are just a few examples of anti-inflammatory spices that can add depth and health benefits to your meals.

Be mindful of cooking methods: Opt for cooking methods that preserve the nutritional value of your ingredients.

Steaming, baking, grilling, and sautéing are healthier alternatives to deep-frying or heavily processing foods.

Stay hydrated: Water plays a vital role in maintaining overall health and reducing inflammation. Aim to drink an adequate amount of water throughout the day and limit sugary beverages.

Prioritize sleep and stress management: Chronic stress and lack of sleep can contribute to inflammation. Prioritize quality sleep and explore stress-management techniques such as meditation, yoga, or engaging in hobbies to support your well-being.

Listen to your body: Each individual's response to food can vary. Pay attention to how your body reacts to certain foods and make adjustments accordingly. Consider consulting with a healthcare professional or registered dietitian for personalized guidance.

By incorporating these practices into your daily routine, you can continue to reap the benefits of an anti-inflammatory lifestyle long after completing the 28-day program outlined in this cookbook. Remember, small changes over time can yield significant results when it comes to your health.

As we bid farewell, it is important to acknowledge the impact of this journey. The 28-Day Prevention Anti-Inflammatory Cookbook was designed not only to provide you with nourishing recipes but also to empower you with knowledge and tools to take control of your health. We hope that this cookbook has sparked a newfound appreciation for the healing power of food and inspired you to make positive choices for yourself and your loved ones.

In closing, let us remember that the journey to optimal health is an ongoing process. While this cookbook provides a solid foundation, it is up to you to continue exploring, experimenting, and discovering new ways to support your well-being. May your path be filled with vibrant, inflammation-fighting meals and a life infused with vitality and vitality.

Thank you for joining us on this transformative journey. Here's to your continued health and wellness!